Better Hearing

Better Hearing

How to Improve Hearing without a Hearing Aid and Treat Tinnitus Naturally

Adam Mills & Instafo

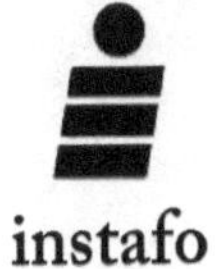

instafo

Copyright © Instafo

All rights reserved.

It is impermissible to reproduce any part of this book without prior consent. All violations will be prosecuted to the fullest extent of the law.

While attempts have been made to verify the information contained within this publication, neither the author nor the publisher assumes any responsibility for errors, omissions, interpretation or usage of the subject matter herein.

This publication contains the opinions and ideas of its author and is intended for informational purpose only. The author and publisher shall in no event be held liable for any loss or other damages incurred from the usage of this publication.

ISBN 978-1-793-40760-3

Printed in the United States of America

First Edition

CONTENTS

Chapter 6: Review and Reflection for Better Hearing

Chapter 7: Resolution and Encouragement for Better Hearing

<u>Chapter 1:</u>

Precaution and Prevention for Better Hearing

Modern Hearing Risk

Imagine <u>not</u> being able to hear the familiar sounds of everyday life: birds singing, music playing, rain falling, and the familiar and comforting voices of your friends and loved ones. That's a frightening thought.

Hearing is one of the vital senses we take for granted.

Thinking about it, perhaps it's time to take better care of your ears, don't you think? That care goes far and beyond just cleaning your ears every now and then, which is important to do. You should also pay attention to the *inside* of your ears. After all, that's where the important stuff happens like hearing, filtering sounds, and helping you decipher voices.

But we live in a world that's not so *"ear friendly."* With all our gadgets and devices, we have become reckless (even though our parents taught us better) and refuse to lower the volume when we watch TV, listen to some tunes, or even put on our headphones. We all know that extremely loud sounds can't be good for our ears, but we seem to ignore it.

Over time, *these habits can damage our hearing*, exposing us to serious hearing loss problems, and even deafness.

Absolute Auditory Awareness

Of course, **taking good care of our ears is the right thing to do.** But it's also important to be aware of other possible causes of hearing loss.

What to watch out for:

- *Head trauma*, possibly caused by a fall or a bump on the head

- *Viruses or diseases* (like meningitis), which are very contagious and deadly if untreated

- *Autoimmune inner ear diseases*, as a result of antibodies and immune cells over-responding and damaging the inner ear.

- *Hereditary hearing loss*, when one or more relatives have had a history of hearing loss

- *Aging*, which is common and perfectly natural as we tend to lose some of our abilities with age

- *Malformation of the inner ear*, which could be something you were born with and obviously had no control over

- *Lack of hygiene*, where people forget to remove ear wax from time to time. An excessive buildup of ear wax can affect your hearing.

On the other hand, if you are careful and take good care of your ears, then you can take advantage of opportunities such as these:

- You won't have to give up your job or be restricted to do certain jobs that rely on your ability to hear.

- You won't risk making mistakes or putting yourself in harm's ways by not hearing certain sounds and noises, like a car horn or someone's shout.

- You will get to enjoy basic conversations with friends without annoying them by asking them to repeat themselves over and over again.

- You will save yourself from the pain that comes with an ear infection, or other hearing diseases.

- And, last but not least, you will not become deaf because of something you could have avoided so easily in the first place.

Complex Interconnected Mechanism

The ability to hear is a complex interconnected mechanism. Sound travels through your ear canal to the eardrum. There, the cochlea receives the sound causing tiny hair cells called stereocilia to vibrate the sound to your brain to be interpreted.

Now let's put this into perspective...

Think about the sounds your car makes when you start the engine or are driving down the road.

The car's headlights are like your eyes because they can help you see when you drive at night. The engine is like your heart because, without it, the car dies. Finally, you can try to diagnose what's wrong with your car if it makes unusual noises when you start the engine, accelerate, hit the brakes, or simply while the engine is running.

If your car is in good condition, the engine and other components will sound smooth and consistent. However, when you don't have enough oil, water for the radiator, or when your battery needs to be charged, the car may make some weird or unusual noises. These noises can be compared to you losing your ability to hear all of a sudden.

When it comes to how your ears process sounds, if a part of your body is not working properly, everything else can soon follow and affect your hearing. That is the beginning sign that you need to start taking better care of yourself.

Basically, trying to distinguish the root cause of your hearing loss is no easy feat as there are many factors involved. But then again, there can be multiple solutions to correcting or fixing your hearing problem, even as simple as changing your diet or massaging the ear, which we will all get into later.

An Important Disclaimer

If you are currently undergoing a medical procedure, or have been prescribed some medication in order to help you with any hearing loss issue, do not stop your treatment. It is important that you follow your doctor's recommendations. The hearing restoration tips we're giving you are not a substitute for your doctor's treatment.

Chapter 2:

Evaluation and Explanation for Better Hearing

The Role of Hearing Frequencies

Are you familiar with the **different frequencies** of hearing? Check out the following audiograms, which are charts that show your hearing ability.

- The *first one*, **Fig.1**, is an example of a <u>speech banana</u> audiogram.

- The *second one*, **Fig.2**, is a <u>regular</u> audiogram showing the **different levels of hearing loss.**

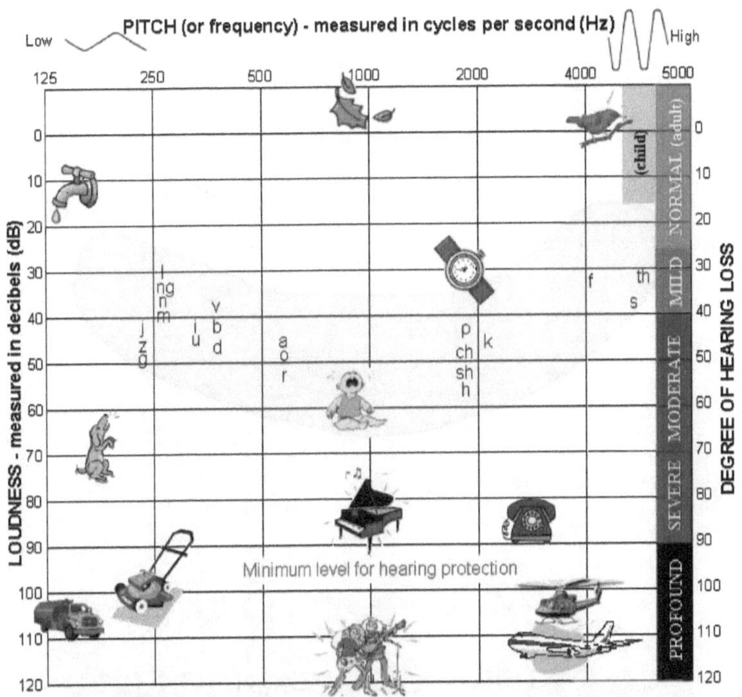

Fig.1. Typical Speech Banana (Ear Community, a charitable nonprofit organization - Microtia and Atresia Support Group)

In this first chart, you have the distinction between **soft** sounds *(from water drops and leaves)*, to **medium** and **moderate noises** *(a baby crying, a dog barking, and the sound* *of a piano)*, to very **heavy noises** *(like music during a concert or an airplane)*.

Each of these noises is represented in terms of their **pitch** (measured in <u>frequency</u>), and in terms of **loudness** (measured in <u>decibels</u>).

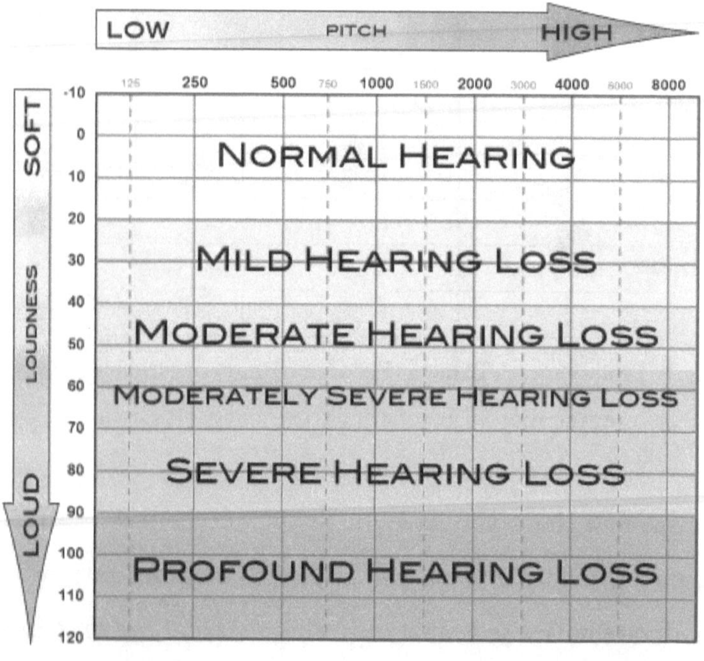

Fig.2. Regular Audiogram (The National Hearing Test)

This second audiogram also follows this logic, but with less detail, where your **level of noise intolerance** is measured *vertically* and *horizontally*.

With both audiograms, the further down (vertically) you go into the graph, the least noise tolerant you become.

Hearing Test: Determine Your Frequency Level

As a first exercise, we would like to give you a small frequency test so that you can define the severity of your hearing loss or whether you suffer from tinnitus or any other hearing problem.

Before you complete this exercise, you should note that tones go from <u>8 Hz</u> all the way up to <u>22,000 Hz</u> (where people <u>over 25</u> are generally not able to hear above <u>15,000 Hz</u>).

According to **The Physics Factbook** (https://hypertextbook.com/facts/2003/ChrisDAmbrose.shtml), a healthy young person hears all sound frequencies from approximately 20Hz to 20,000 Hz.

The <u>video linked below</u> includes a series of tones ranging from <u>20 Hz</u> to <u>20,000 Hz</u>. The aim of the exercise is to listen to each tone and note when your hearing cuts out.

Start the exercise by **turning the volume <u>down</u>** on your headphones or speakers and **then gradually turn it to a safe level** *(not too high)*. Overall, if you need to *increase the volume* as the *frequency increases*, then you may have a **hearing problem**.

Take a listen: www.youtube.com/watch?v=y7ocOKvfoZg

(Note: There are similar tests like this out there. You can find a lot of them online. Just do a search for "hearing frequency test.")

When you reach **your limit** *(when the sound cuts out)*, pause the video and write down that <u>last frequency</u> you were able to hear. Then find that frequency in either one of the charts above. Remember that the frequency or pitch is listed at the top of each chart. The left side indicates decibels.

<u>Decibels</u> designate the **level of volume** you can tolerate depending on the <u>frequency</u> you are hearing. *A little confused?* Take your time looking at the charts, and they will start to make sense.

Got it? Good. Go do that now, then come back for your result.

Your Result: Where You Fall in the Hearing Range

After figuring out the frequency that you can *hear up to*, find the conclusion below that best describes your current hearing condition:

- If you are between <u>0</u> to <u>25 dB</u>, your hearing faculties are considered **normal**. You probably have decent habits when it comes to noises. Chances are, you don't sleep with earphones on, and when you start to feel uncomfortable with loud music, you simply turn it off or lower the volume. Hooray for you! But definitely continue onward because we have some very interesting information on how to delay the loss of your hearing abilities with age.

- If you are between <u>30</u> and <u>70 dB</u>, you may have **some hearing issues** where you can't tolerate loud sounds for too long, or you are already showing signs of someone who easily gets irritated by minimal sounds because your ears are not trained enough to drown out certain unnecessary sounds. You should be alerted by this sensitivity to (even) minor sounds since it might be a sign that your hearing is in distress from too much exposure to loud noises. Take note concerning the "physical exercises" and the ones involving white noises (we'll explain those a little later) as they can help you reinforce your hearing muscles and organs and help you ignore unnecessary noises.

- If you are between <u>70</u> and <u>120 dB</u>, you may have **severe** to **profound hearing issues**. You may suffer from recurring episodes of tinnitus, headaches due to loud or sharp noises, hyperacusis, etc. You may be wearing some type of hearing aid to help you listen and recognize noises, and you may be the type of individual who needs people to speak louder in order for you to hear them properly. Take note and follow the advice given throughout.

A Natural Process

Regardless of where you fall in the hearing range, it's perfectly normal that we all lose some of our hearing abilities as we get older. So don't be alarmed if you haven't been to an audiologist for a long time or have never been for that matter, and this is the first time that you've discovered that you have some hearing loss. (Obviously, for a more accurate result, you should see an audiologist.)

The majority of the population doesn't regularly get their hearing checked like they do, for example, with regular eye exams. So they become anxious when they realize that they can no longer hear as they used to as a kid, which nobody can.

The great news is that you have taken a conscious effort and desire into protecting and preserving your hearing for the long haul, and with the potential to make it better than where it is now, with natural techniques.

So, you are already that much ahead of the oblivious herd.

<u>Chapter 3:</u>

Nutrition and Supplements for Better Hearing

Common Hearing Disorders

Some of the most common hearing problems are <u>tinnitus</u> and <u>hyperacusis.</u> These problems are often associated with our lifestyle choices.

- **Tinnitus** is an uncomfortable sensation of sound you get in your ears. Do you ever suddenly hear a <u>ringing</u>, <u>hissing</u> or <u>buzzing</u> in your ears when there are no external sounds present? Then you may be among the approximately 17 percent of the U.S.

population that suffers from tinnitus. This is often a sign of hearing loss, the impact of a recent head injury, tension in an ear muscle or possibly the side effect of a prescribed or unprescribed drug.

- **Hyperacusis** is lack of tolerance for loud or sometimes routine noises. Does it sometimes seem like routine sounds like a running faucet, an appliance, or a car engine are far louder than they should be? Then you may suffer from hyperacusis. It is often caused by lifestyle choices, for example, the overexposure to loud noises for a long time.

Renowned doctor, Mao Shing Ni (popularly known as *Dr. Mao*), is the co-founder of the California-based **Tao of Wellness**, an award-winning center for health and traditional Chinese medicine including nutrition, acupuncture, and anti-aging. Dr. Mao is the inspiration for most of the natural remedies that we will discuss.

<u>Note</u>: We will start by working *from the inside out* with our hearing health, and then get into the more *external, hands-on aspects* later. If nutrition or supplements don't interest you all that much, you *may skip ahead* to the sections dealing with practical "<u>hearing exercises</u>" and "<u>hearing application</u>." However, it would be worth your wild to at least know what should go into your body to support healthy hearing.

So now, when it comes to things you should drink and eat that can improve your hearing every day, Dr. Mao recommends these upcoming things.

Spicy Ginger Tea

What you will need:
- 1 tablespoon of dried oregano
- 1 tablespoon of cilantro
- 1 tablespoon of rosemary
- 1 tablespoon of sage
- 1 tablespoon of cinnamon

- 3 slices of fresh ginger *(Ginger has been used for medicinal purposes, mainly in China.)*
- 4 cups of water

Preparation: Boil all the ingredients for <u>15 minutes</u>. Let it sit for 30 seconds.

How to use it: Drink three cups a day, preferably in the morning, after lunch and at night before you go to bed. Think of these cups of ginger tea as hearing wellness shots that you will have to take three times a day, for at least three weeks. Meanwhile, refrain from exposure to loud noises and anything else that may affect your hearing during this natural healing phase.

Bone Marrow Soup

What you will need:

- Some organic sheep bones or calf bones
- 8 cups of water
- 1/3 cup of black beans

- Kidney beans
- Adzuki beans
- 2 diced carrots
- 2 diced celery stalks
- 1 sliced onion
- 1/2 cup of dried seaweed
- 1 teaspoon of turmeric
- 1 teaspoon of cumin
- 1 teaspoon of black pepper

Preparation: Boil all these ingredients, except for the spices, together. Then season with the turmeric, cumin, and black pepper. No salt is needed.

How to use it: You should eat this soup four times a month if you want to see results. Of course, if you want to see long-lasting results, you will also have to make some lifestyle adjustments, like avoiding loud noises, avoiding certain drugs that can affect your hearing, and any other high-risk activity.

Assignment: Add Beneficial Nutrients to Your Diet

Here's your assignment for the next few weeks to a month.

- Prepare the ginger tea following the instructions mentioned. Drink three cups a day as your daily hearing wellness shots.

- After three weeks, document your hearing improvements. Throughout this process, be sure to avoid loud noises and any risky activity. Make sure you test your hearing improvement by perhaps checking your hearing weaknesses. For example, if there are certain noises you usually can't hear, have trouble distinguishing various noises, or constantly have to ask people to repeat themselves because you didn't hear them, make a note of how well you have improved over these three weeks.

- After these first three weeks, see if you can incorporate the ginger tea into your daily routine. If you are a regular coffee drinker, replace one or more of your regular cups with a cup of this ginger tea.

- You can make and eat the bone marrow soup once every month from now on.

By following these suggestions, you can improve your hearing and overall health.

Vital Supplements

Taking supplements can be a great way to fight hearing loss. The interesting thing about this is that you don't necessarily have to avoid certain areas where there are a lot of noises.

In a way, taking supplements can be viewed as helping to reinforce your hearing muscles and to restore a more wholesome hearing.

Here are some interesting and effective supplements to consider:

- **N-acetylcysteine (NAL 500 mg)**: It is essentially used to prevent rashes, urticaria, and itchiness, among other things. So what does that have to do with your hearing? Well, there's an important antioxidant known as glutathione. Dr. Frank Shallenberger, a Nevada-based anti-aging and natural remedy expert, suggests that people with hearing problems often lack that antioxidant. He says glutathione will not only help repair ear damage caused by loud noises, but it will also boost the body's production of glutathione. It's like a two-for-one special!

- **Folate (folic acid 400 micrograms)**: Maybe you've heard of folate by its other name, folic acid. It's a B vitamin found in some of the foods we eat, and it's typically used by pregnant women since it helps combat anemia. But you don't have to be pregnant, or even a woman, to get hearing benefits from folic acid. A study presented in 2009 at the annual meeting at the American Academy of Otolaryngology-Head and Neck Surgery Foundation (AAO-HNSF) showed that men over the age of 60 who have a high intake of foods and supplements high in folates have a 20 percent decrease in risk of losing their hearing abilities. *Now that's an easy way to protect your hearing!*

- **Carotenoids (1,000 mg)**: Carotenoids are organic pigments mostly produced by plants and algae, as well as several bacteria and fungi. *Consuming algae, bacteria, and fungi?!* Don't worry, you won't be licking the walls of a dirty sink! Carotenoids are recommended as supplements to help with recovering from hearing loss because they are known to protect against oxidative stress in the cochlea. They help prevent free radical damage, improve blood flow and also improve homocysteine metabolism.

- **Lipo-flavonoid**: This supplement is mostly recommended for people who suffer exclusively from tinnitus. Remember, that's the unusual ringing or other sounds in your ears. Lipo-flavonoid supplement is a concentrated extract of lemon peel, ascorbic acid (or vitamin C), eriodyctiol glycoside, choline, and inositol. For satisfactory results, you should take it for at least six months.

Natural-Boosting Herbs

A list of supplements wouldn't be complete if we didn't include the more natural herbs. They have been used for centuries, way before we started synthesizing their components for modern medicine.

Again, Dr. Mao as well as pharmacists like Scott Gavura in Ontario, Canada recommend two very popular herbs and traditional Chinese herbs:

- **Gingko Biloba** can help stabilize hearing loss by increasing capillary blood circulation.

- **Hawthorn Berry** originated from Europe but is also grown in Asia and North America, and can help with blood flow in preventing hearing loss.

- **Traditional Chinese Herbs** like include Rehmannia, wild yam, schisandra, Asian cornelian, and magnetite support healthy hearing.

And yes, they help combat deafness. So don't discount adding these herbs into your life.

Dietary Supplement Incorporation

All of these supplements and herbs can be readily found at your local pharmacy or online and be used as extracts for your tea or water or be taken as convenient powder capsules or pills.

You can also find them combined into one another, such as the "ginkgo" and "hawthorn" both mixed together in one capsule form. Same for most of the traditional Chinese herbs for hearing which can be found formulated under the Chinese name "Er Long Zuo Ci Pian."

Let's be honest, many people who attempt to take vitamins or other supplements regularly don't always stick to their routine. It's similar to going on a diet. Many of us end up cheating on the diet or not following it consistently.

To make it easier for you, put a daily dose of whatever supplements that you're going to take each on a small plate lined up prominently on your table or counter, like a buffet that you are going to finish throughout the day. Ideally, you would want to do this the night before or in the morning as you prepare breakfast and the rest of your day.

Having some tangible visual display out in the open can help remind and ensure that you take your daily vitamins.

<u>Important</u>: Of course, always talk to your doctor first regarding any supplements you intend to take, as combining some supplements at the same time or into your diet can have an adverse effect. Make sure that you follow the <u>UL</u> or **tolerable upper intake level** of these nutrients in order to avoid cases of overdose and any other complications. If you have any questions about the prescribed dosage written on the package, be sure to talk to your doctor.

Assignment: Set Up Your Supplemental Routine

As an experiment each morning or the night before, try setting up the supplements that you're taking each on a small plate all prominently displayed like freshly cooked meals that will go to waste and leave you with guilt if you don't finish them.

Do this as a routine for at least three months and document the changes you observe by stating how clearly you can hear sounds, and how signs of migraines or pain to the ear have now decreased or completely stopped, etc.

Remember to adopt better habits when it comes to noises. As we said earlier, adjusting your environment is also important to your healing process. So start listening to music or watching TV at a lower volume and clean your ears regularly. The proof will be in the results.

Chapter 4:

Exercising and Conditioning for Better Hearing

Workout for the Hearing

Sometimes it's hard to exercise...but we're not asking you to do pushups or jumping jacks. We're talking about exercising your ears.

Huh, what? That's right! As unorthodox as that may sound, there are exercises that you can do to strengthen and enforce your hearing.

Continue onward to learn about these fascinating methods as natural alternatives.

Ear Exercise: Earlobes Tug

This ear exercise expands and opens up your ear canal and auditory tube (the inner-nasal area to the eardrum) that may be clogged and needs the tension or pressure to be released.

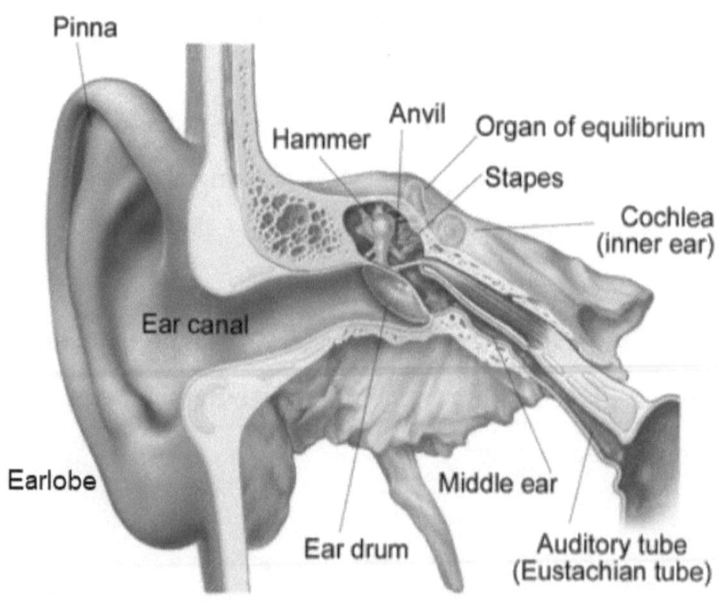

1. Take your thumb and index finger and grab your bottom earlobe. You can do one or both ears at the same time.

2. Squeeze it and rub in a circular motion for about <u>30 seconds</u>.

3. Then pull the earlobe in an out-upward <u>45-degree angle</u> direction. They should be <u>5</u> quick tug pulls. Don't pull too hard like you're trying to pull your ear off, but make sure you feel the *tightness* behind your ear per each quick tug.

This may seem very simple, but give this a try and you should notice a difference in how your ear feels as well as in your hearing.

Hearing Exercise 1: Imaginary Drums

Do you remember when you were a kid and you were told that if you hold a seashell up to your ear you could magically hear the ocean? Well, that is actually the inner noise your human body naturally makes, which sounds something like a windy drumming sound.

Our first exercise consists of covering your ears and simulating that drumming sound while breathing. The purpose is to synchronize the brain with this inner sound that the ear perceives (or recognizes) without external interference.

This is extremely beneficial for those who suffer from tinnitus by masking or overriding the tinnitus sound with the unnoticeable natural sound that your body makes.

1. In a quiet place, and preferably while sitting down, place both hands over your ears. Do not press too hard,

as the lack of air will create the sensation of your hand being pulled into your ear (kind of like a suction, which can be very uncomfortable especially if you are already experiencing pain in your ears).

2. With your hands placed over your ears, breathe in and out and mentally record the sound it makes, which is like the sound of an imaginary drum. Do this for <u>60 seconds</u>.

3. After <u>60 seconds</u>, remove your hands from your ears, breathe in and out, then repeat the process a second time for another <u>60 seconds</u>.

Hearing Exercise 2: Imaginary Bells

The second exercise consists of simulating the sounds of bells by combining breathing, covering your ears, and this time, biting down. Here's how to do it:

1. Once again, in a quiet place, cover your ears with minimal pressure.

2. Bite down by slightly closing your jaw and breathe in and out through your nose.

3. Repeat the word *"one"* with your mouth closed. The *"one"* sound you produce with your mouth closed will sound like a church bell being struck by the bell's inside clapper. You should also feel some vibrations around your left and right temporal bone areas where your ears are located. Do this slowly for a total of <u>10 bell sounds</u>.

4. Take your hands off your ears and breathe in and out, allowing your ears to relax.

5. Do this whole process one more time.

These two hearing exercises are usually best done at night before going to sleep because that's usually when there are fewer noises around the house. Doing it at night will also give your ears the time to rest after a good exercise and allow you to wake up the next morning with sharper and fresh hearing.

Nevertheless, do them at whatever time is the quietest for you. Just spare yourself <u>three</u> to <u>five minutes</u> in order to perform either or both of these exercises.

Ear Protection Practice

This isn't really an exercise but a **best practice**. This is important, so listen up (*pun intended!*).

Always protect your ears with **earplugs** when you are going to be in a noisy environment. This includes concerts, major sporting events or other public gatherings, as well as when you are using loud machinery like your lawn mower. Earplugs are cheap and easy to find at pharmacies, supermarkets, or online.

- There are many kinds that reduce the level of decibels. The *foam ones* are the most popular, but you can also try the *silicone ones* that swimmers use.

- There are even fancier earplugs that allow you to hear regular sounds like conversation but will only *reduce louder noises* above a <u>certain decibel</u>. For instance, you can hear a regular conversation as usual as if you weren't using earplugs, but when you go outside and somebody honks a loud horn, that sound will be reduced to protect your hearing. These are the type of earplugs that musicians use. They are more expensive, but you don't have to be a rock star to afford them.

Just use whatever earplugs you're most comfortable with.

Chapter 5:

Advanced Application and Alternative Alteration for Better Hearing

Tea Tree Oil Massage

Now we shall move on with additional practical application.

First, going back to one of Dr. Mao's recommendations.

Any time you want to relax, give yourself a tea tree oil massage. It's great for your ears and also nice right before you go to bed.

What you will need:

- 3 drops of tea tree oil

- 2 tablespoons of olive oil

- 1 tablespoon of colloidal vinegar

- 1 tablespoon of apple cider vinegar

How to use it: Mix all the oils together then warm the mixture for about 60 to 90 seconds. Be careful! You don't want it to get too hot. Massage the oil around your ears. If you feel any pain, you can dip a piece of cotton into the oil and then massage the affected area or put the oily piece of cotton directly on it for five minutes. Continue doing this for two days. Once again, avoid any risky behavior or habit that may prevent this method from working effectively. Stay away from noises and risky activities, like the ones where you may get a head injury.

Acupuncture for Hearing Loss

Let's get right to the *point* about **acupuncture**. Scientific evidence proves how acupuncture can help your hearing.

Check out this study by medical experts at the Chinese PLA General Hospital and Daqing Hospital of Traditional Chinese Medicine (*"Efficacy and safety of acupuncture therapy for nerve deafness: a meta-analysis of randomized controlled trials."* Int J Clin Exp Med 8, no. 2 (2015): 2614-2620): www.ncbi.nlm.nih.gov/pmc/articles/PMC4402856/

The study concluded that acupuncture is a very effective way to improve the hearing of patients with nerve deafness. The doctors recommend that the treatment is combined with medication. *So if you are currently taking some medication to help with hearing loss, you can keep taking it while incorporating acupuncture as well.*

Regarding the common ringing, beeping, or buzzing symptom in your ears, tinnitus, there is no cure for it *according* to most western doctors other than to learn to ignore it. But in the eastern part of the world, acupuncture is a plausible treatment method depending on the cause, as one study has shown: (*"The effects of acupuncture on the inner ear originated tinnitus."* J Res Med Sci. 2011 Sep; 16(9):

1217–1223):

www.ncbi.nlm.nih.gov/pmc/articles/PMC3430048/

If you are interested in acupuncture, the best thing to do is find a **medical doctor** who is also trained in *Traditional Chinese Medicine* and is a licensed acupuncturist. This way you'll combine both western and eastern medicine. You can find such a doctor by asking around or visiting a medical website like ZocDoc.com.

You can also try **acupressure** at home with two exercises, one focused *on your feet*, and the other focused on the nerves *around your ears*. Here's how.

Foot Acupressure

You are probably wondering, why apply acupressure to your foot when we are talking about the ears? This is based on the therapy of **reflexology** where stimulating certain points of the body can relieve problems in other parts of the body.

Foot Reflexology Chart

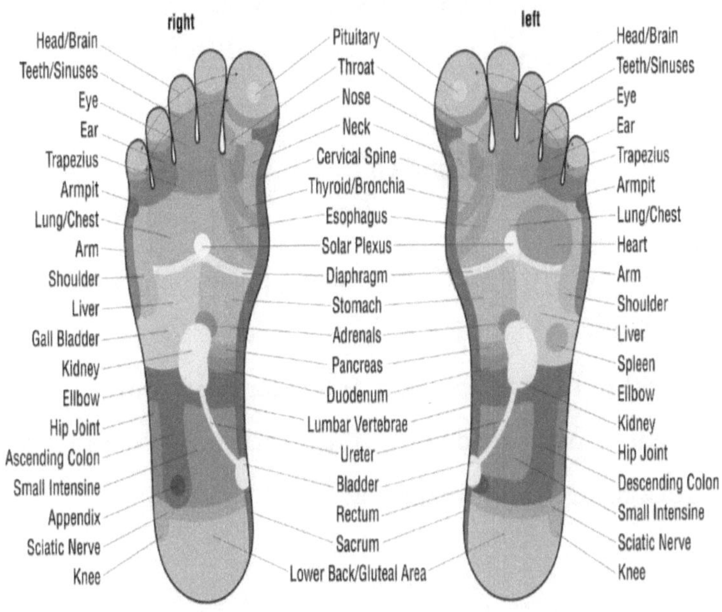

1. Begin by finding the **acupoints** for the ear on the tip and base of the *last two toes*. Refer to the chart above.

2. Start with your right foot. Apply some pressure steadily for <u>two minutes</u> with your right thumb until you feel soreness.

3. Now repeat this process with your left foot. Make sure your movements are swift and that you remain calm and focused by breathing slowly.

Do-It-Yourself Ear Acupressure

1. Locate the acupoint **"listening palace"** also known in acupuncture practice as **SI-19**, which is the area located right in front of the right or left ear canal (in the depression formed when you slightly open your mouth). See SI-19 in the image below.

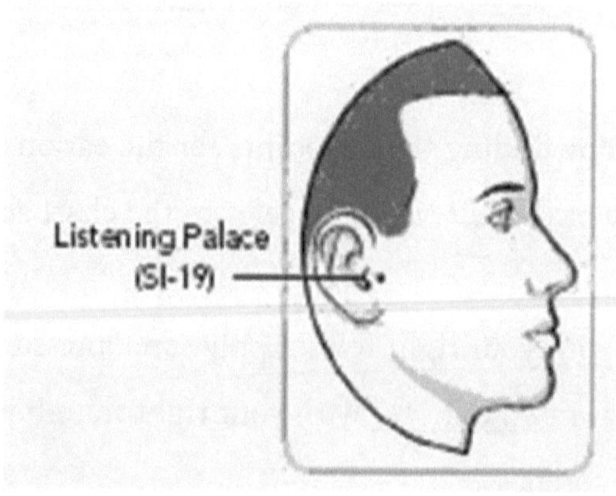

2. Start with your right ear. Apply a steady pressure for 2 minutes to the area with your index finger until soreness begins.

3. Repeat the process with your left ear, with swift movements, and concentration.

Self-acupressure is a way to heal your hearing and also help with blood flow. By following these exercises, you can help rejuvenate and preserve your hearing for a long time.

White Noise Masking

Condition yourself to filter out unwanted noises with the help of white noises.

Think about how your brain works when you are distracted. Ultimately, your brain will focus on the one thing you've got your mind on. In some cases, you can't even hear what a person a few feet away from you is saying because you're so focused.

That is what happens with **white noises** because as audiologist Tracy Saunders says, white noises help the brain focus on one sound *(suppressing any background sound)*. She encourages using white noises *(especially as a sleeping aid)* but by monitoring the sound *(with the sound set at a low level)*.

White noise can be very soothing, especially for people suffering from disruptive conditions like tinnitus, because it helps the ear drown out the uncomfortable sound (thanks to the frequencies released from the white noises).

There are **different types of white sounds,** and they can consist of *frequency sounds*, or sounds of *nature* (river, rain, wind, etc.). What you should do with these sounds is get accustomed to them, register them in your mind, and replay them during the day when faced with loud or distracting noises (cars, voices, music, etc.) that you can't always control.

Here's how you should use white noises to ignore sounds and reduce the impact of tinnitus:

1. Use a white noise sound like the one in this video (or search for *"binaural beats white noise"*): www.youtube.com/watch?v=hJsp-1aKTgE.

2. Focus on the sound, close your eyes and breathe slowly.

3. Listen to the sound for about <u>30 minutes</u>. You will feel calmer all of the sudden, almost like you are falling asleep.

4. When you reach close to the <u>30-minute</u> mark, turn off the sound.

5. Your hearing should now feel slightly altered for the better as you readjust yourself back into the present moment.

This application not only helps you listen more attentively to things but also blocks out unwanted noises.

Using white noise doesn't mean you have to be confined to an undisturbed meditative state for 30 minutes. Another way you can use it is to have it as background noise to mask unwanted sound. The white noise doesn't have to be a professionally-produced audio recording with binaural beats; any natural calming sound that has a nice steady rhythm to it like that of a refrigerator, fan, air conditioner, air purifier, *etc.*, will do.

This benefits those who have trouble working in a quiet environment or at night trying to sleep due to the inner-ear noise they experience from their tinnitus. So, having something as simple as a fan running as background noise can help people focus at work or go to sleep when everything is silent.

Body Realignment for Hearing Readjustment

In some cases, hearing issues can be fixed by readjusting your body's neck posture, facial muscles, or jaw alignment.

To figure out if that is the case for you, do you notice any fluctuation in your hearing when you move your neck, mouth, face, etc.?

- For example, if you have tinnitus, whenever you yawn or open your mouth as wide as possible, does the tinnitus subside? Then your case of tinnitus may be related to some misalignment of your mouth or jaw affecting the temporal bone area around your ear, commonly known as "somatic tinnitus." If so, correcting your jaw by seeing an orthodontist or oral surgeon may be advised.

- If your tinnitus tends to be louder first thing in the morning after lying down in bed all night but it diminishes or disappears throughout the day, then changing your sleeping position or seeing a chiropractor to correct your neck or back posture could provide relief.

- If whenever you move your neck to a certain direction, you notice that the tone of what you hear changes, then stretching or massaging your neck to loosen tension in the "sternocleidomastoid muscle" that connects behind the ear may help balance your hearing.

This is one of the biggest reasons why hearing issues such as tinnitus are so complex to solve because there are different variables involved for every unique individual's case.

Only you know your body best. So listen to it, and it will guide you to better health.

Hygienic Hearing Health

Lastly, we would like to say that cleaning your ears regularly is also important if you want to preserve your hearing abilities.

You've probably heard warnings about not using Q-tips or other cotton swabs because they tend to push the wax deeper inside the ear cavity. That's good advice to adhere to. You should not stick anything into the ear canal.

But if you can't use a cotton swab, how can you clean inside your ears?

Never fear, there are other ways to clean them.

- You can wash the external part of your ears with a washcloth anytime you wash your face or take a shower.

- For cleaning the inside, you can place a few drops of mineral oil, baby oil, glycerin or wax-removing drops in the ear in order to loosen the wax and make it easier to come out. It's okay to repeat the process at least every <u>five</u> to <u>seven</u> days. You may even notice improved hearing once you get the wax under control.

Chapter 6:

Review and Reflection for Better Hearing

Now that we've shared new ways for you to protect and improve your hearing, it's time to put what you've learned into action. As a review, give each of these exercises a try, and be sure to document your results.

Review Exercise 1: Relaxing Rain

1. Go to a quiet place and listen to this natural sound of raindrops for 30 minutes:

www.youtube.com/watch?v=jX6kn9_U8qk

2. While you're listening, be sure to breathe slowly and release any tension. *Relaxing, isn't it?*

3. After a while, you may feel so cozy and comfortable that you'll want to doze off. This is an indication that the sound has "tamed" your mind and that it will stick there for a while because of the comfort it brings. When that happens, you can stop listening, take a deep breath, and go about the rest of your day.

4. Whether you are at a public place, at the office, at the store, or wherever, listening to white noise can readjust your hearing to be more intently focused rather than be distracted by the background noises or (if you have tinnitus) the sound in your head.

<u>Self-Reflection:</u>

- How effective is it for you to block out "bothersome noises" ever since you've started listening to white noise?

Review Exercise 2: Calming Bells

1. Find a quiet place and cover your ears (remember, no excessive pressure).

2. While breathing through your nose and biting down, repeat the word *"one"* slowly <u>10 times</u> to mimic the sound of a church bell, then stop, breathe, and repeat.

3. Complete <u>two cycles</u> of this whole process.

<u>Self-Reflection</u>:

- How easy is it for you to better distinguish certain noises?

- How fluid are sounds now, ever since you've started doing this?

- Can you hear noises from a farther distance?

Review Exercise 3: Dietary Display

Whatever supplements or nutrients that you're adding to your regimen, try preparing them ahead of time each on a small plate with their proper daily dosage prominently displayed like a combo platter to remind you to take them.

<u>Self-Reflection:</u>

- Do you find doing this makes taking supplements much easier and faster?

- Do you notice any change so far in your hearing since you started taking the supplements?

Review Exercise 4: One-Month Change

Try using ginger tea as a remedy to combat hearing loss for one month. At the same time, you should watch TV with a lower volume. Do not use headphones or earbuds when you want to listen to music. Do not yell when you speak, or behave in any way that could damage your hearing.

One-Month Self-Reflection:

- How fluid are the sounds now?

- Can you pick up and hone in on more sounds now (such as multiple background sounds)?

- Are any sounds that were previously unpleasant or irritating to you now tolerable?

Chapter 7:

Resolution and Encouragement for Better Hearing

The Ever-Increasing Harm on the Hearing

We have now reached the end. It's time to wrap everything up so you can take what you have learned and incorporate it into your life.

Losing your hearing can be scary for anybody. With all the gadgets and modern technologies we have, it seems that we are exposed to hearing risks more now than ever before. Think about your headphones, earbuds, powerful sound systems, and more.

Technology and entertainment can be good, but there are risks involved with such loud sounds. It is especially problematic for kids and teens because, with all these gadgets, they are already adopting bad hearing habits at an early age. Some people even listen to loud music on headphones when they go to sleep. (*Wouldn't you rather listen to calming white noise?*)

Then combine that with the natural decrease in hearing ability that we face as we get older. So, what will happen to the younger generations who use these "high risk" headphones so early in their lives? It turns out most of them are at risk of becoming partially or totally deaf way earlier than the generations before them. That is indeed a very frightening thought.

About 20 years ago, it was a common belief that hearing loss was irreversible. For that reason, doctors prescribed certain medication to try to mitigate the symptoms. But with prescription drugs, there are always potential side effects.

The Cutting-Edge Breakthrough on the Horizon

The good news is, with a growing interest in alternative healing methods, people now have natural remedy options, such as: making ginger tea infusions, using herbs rich in antioxidants like hawthorn berries and gingko biloba, or simply training your ears to become more sensitive to certain sounds or to ignore undesirable sounds through the use of white noise.

And don't forget, there is traditional Chinese medicine like acupuncture to alleviate hearing issues, as well as great promise in the future coming from modern science like the possibility of re-growing your ear hair cells to eliminate hearing loss for good (straight from Harvard: https://news.harvard.edu/gazette/story/2017/03/replacing-damaged-hair-cells-may-help-treat-hearing-loss/).

Think of it this way, back then optical eyewear like glasses were the only means to improve your eyesight. But wearing glasses can be a burden, not to mention if you lose them. Then along came the advancement of LASIK eye surgery where the solution to eye correction was no longer a band-aid over the problem.

We are getting closer to the same point where wearing hearing aids will no longer be the band-aid solution to improving your hearing. With the never-ending breakthroughs, we might one day finally be able to restore natural hearing completely.

In the meantime, while waiting for science to work miracles, you can start protecting, preserving, and improving your hearing abilities now and use them for much longer than ever before.

Doesn't that *pleasantly sound* like something worth doing *to your ears*? Of course it is, otherwise why else would you still be here making it this far? So start today! It will be well worth it!